Yoga Therapy

Healing the Body, Relieving Pain

James E. Green

TABLE OF CONTENT

INTRODUCTION

In the hectic cacophony of contemporary life, when stress, worry, and physical problems have grown widespread, there exists an old and deep treatment — Yoga Therapy. Far beyond the world of popular workout regimens, Yoga Therapy is a comprehensive route to healing and well-being, weaving together the ancient knowledge of yoga with contemporary therapeutic ideas. It is a transforming journey that explores the delicate link between the body, mind, and soul, giving a sanctuary of hope for individuals seeking healing, regeneration, and self-discovery.

Story:
Once, in a busy metropolis, there lived a lady called Maya, who found herself embroiled in the constant maelstrom of duties and expectations. Her days were occupied with long hours at a demanding profession, managing domestic chores, and battling with the weight of unresolved emotional issues. Each night, she lay awake, a prisoner of her racing thoughts and the physical strain that had braided its way into her existence.

One fateful day, as she travelled through the city streets, overwhelmed by the weight of her problems, she came onto a little, inconspicuous yoga class nestled away in an alley. Intrigued, Maya stepped inside, and there, in the peacefulness of the studio, she met a knowledgeable yoga therapist called Ravi.

Ravi exhibited a deep sense of serenity and compassion that quickly put Maya at rest. As they sat together, Ravi listened closely to Maya's narrative, the words tumbling out like long-held secrets. He knew the enormous load she bore, the grief that had sunk deep inside her heart, and the outward signs of her inner distress.

With a soft grin, Ravi added, "Maya, the practice of yoga therapy goes beyond the surface of the body; it digs into the centre of your being, aiming to untie the knots that bind you. Through breath, movement, and awareness, we may journey together towards healing and change."

Intrigued by Ravi's statements, Maya decided to start on this new road of yoga treatment. Week after week, she came to the studio, peeling back the layers of her inner world, led by Ravi's firm hand and compassionate attitude. Slowly, she learned to abandon her fears, release the grasp of the past, and embrace the present moment with compassion and acceptance.

As she went further into the practice of yoga therapy, Maya felt the shift taking root inside her. The physical tightness that had chained her body started to fade, replaced by a wonderful sensation of comfort and lightness. In the calm of her thoughts, clarity dawned like a soft dawn, revealing the route ahead.

Through the practice of breathwork, Maya found a shelter of serenity and quiet. With each deliberate breath and exhale, she rooted herself in the now, free from the grips of past regrets and future fears.

And so, the days grew into weeks, and the weeks became months. Maya's experience with yoga therapy became a monument to the persistence of the human spirit, a hymn to the transformational power of self-awareness and compassion.

One evening, as the sun dropped below the horizon, throwing a warm light onto the city, Maya stood at the shore of a quiet lake. At that moment, she recognized that the weights she had bore had become stepping stones on her road to recovery and empowerment. Through the discipline of yoga therapy, she regained her life, embracing her inner power and finding consolation in the depths of her own heart.

Maya's experience is simply one of the numerous narratives weaved into the fabric of yoga therapy's significant influence. It is a monument to the ongoing power of an ancient practice that transcends time and culture, giving a refuge of hope and regeneration to all who seek its embrace. With each breath, each mindful movement, and each moment of self-reflection, the transforming journey of yoga therapy continues, weaving its magic into the lives of those who dare to embark upon it.

THE ROLE OF THE YOGA THERAPIST

FOUNDATIONS OF YOGA

Yoga, an ancient practice that started in the mythical region of India, has transcended time and boundaries to become a worldwide path towards harmony, inner serenity, and self-realisation. At its foundation, yoga is not only a physical workout regimen but a deep philosophy that knits together the body, mind, and spirit, giving a holistic approach to well-being.

The origins of yoga may be traced back over 5,000 years to the ancient books of the Vedas and Upanishads. It was within these ancient scriptures that the core ideas of yoga were first established, establishing a way of life that embraced ethical behaviour, self-discipline, and spiritual insight.

The Eight Limbs of Yoga:
Central to the basis of yoga is the concept of the Eight Limbs of Yoga, as explained by the sage Patanjali in the Yoga Sutras. These eight limbs give complete guidance to living a purposeful and meaningful life, embracing both the physical and philosophical components of yoga.

Yamas (Restraints): The Yamas are ethical rules that regulate one's conduct towards oneself and others. They include non-violence (ahimsa), honesty (satya), non-stealing (asteya), moderation (brahmacharya), and non-possessiveness (aparigraha).

Niyamas (Observances): The Niyamas are activities that cultivate self-discipline and inner observation. They include purity (saucha), contentment (santosha), self-discipline (tapas), self-study (svadhyaya), and submission to a higher power (ishvara pranidhana).

Asanas (Postures): Asanas refers to the physical postures done in yoga. Beyond their physical advantages, they are designed to prepare the body and mind for meditation and spiritual investigation.

Pranayama (Breath Control): Pranayama incorporates breathwork methods that teach conscious control and awareness of the breath. It acts as a bridge between the physical and spiritual worlds, soothing the mind and vitalizing the body.

Pratyahara (Withdrawal of the Senses): Pratyahara is the practice of going within by withdrawing the senses from outward distractions. It prepares the mind for deeper stages of meditation and self-reflection.

Dharana (Concentration): Dharana entails concentrating the attention on a single point or object. It cultivates constant focus, preparing the door for meditation.

Dhyana (Meditation): Dhyana is the condition of continuous contemplation when the mind is entirely engrossed in the topic of meditation. It leads to a deep feeling of inner serenity and heightened self-awareness.

Samadhi (Union): Samadhi is the ultimate objective of yoga, indicating a condition of transcendence and oneness with the global mind. It is a state of great awareness and happiness.

Beyond the Eight Limbs, yoga's core concept encompasses the awareness of the interdependence of all living creatures and the realisation of the divine nature inside each person. This awareness lays the foundation for the practice of compassion, kindness, and non-judgment towards others and oneself.

In conclusion, the roots of yoga go beyond physical postures; they incorporate a deep philosophy that has led people toward self-realisation for millennia. The Eight Limbs of Yoga give a complete route toward harmony, inner calm, and spiritual enlightenment. As yoga continues to change and adapt in the contemporary world, its timeless principles remain a source of deep knowledge and inspiration, allowing people of all backgrounds to embark on a transforming journey of self-discovery and inner growth.

UNDERSTANDING YOGA: PHILOSOPHY AND PRACTICE

Yoga practice involves a varied variety of methods and disciplines that address the physical, mental, and spiritual elements of the person. While the physical postures, known as asanas, are undoubtedly the most prominent feature of yoga in the contemporary world, they are merely one facet of a holistic practice.

Asanas: The physical postures of yoga are meant to promote strength, flexibility, and balance in the body. They also serve as a technique to prepare the body for meditation and inner investigation. Each asana is accompanied by attentive breathing, helping practitioners to be completely present in the moment.

Pranayama: Pranayama, or breath control, incorporates numerous breathing methods that promote the flow of life force energy (prana) inside the body. Pranayama techniques quiet the mind, decrease tension, and generate a feeling of relaxation and clarity.

Meditation: Meditation is a cornerstone of yoga practice, giving a technique to quiet the mind, enhance inner awareness, and reach a state of profound inner calm.

Through meditation, practitioners explore the depths of awareness and tap into their inner knowledge.

Yoga Nidra: Yoga Nidra, also known as yogic sleep, is a guided relaxation method that generates a condition of profound rest and regeneration. It lets the body and mind relieve stress and tension, facilitating deep physical and emotional healing.

Mindfulness: Mindfulness is a fundamental aspect of yoga practice, urging people to be completely present in each moment without judgement. Mindful awareness goes beyond the mat into everyday life, generating a feeling of clarity, appreciation, and compassion.

The Integration of Philosophy and Practice:
Understanding yoga as a concept and implementing it through practice is a joyful and transforming path. The philosophy of yoga offers a guiding light, integrating meaning and depth into the practice. As practitioners expand their knowledge of the interconnection of all life and the divinity within, they infuse their practice with a feeling of sanctity and respect.

Through the combination of theory and practice, yoga becomes more than simply physical exercise; it becomes a deep examination of self, a voyage of self-discovery, and a route towards inner peace and spiritual enlightenment.

In conclusion, knowing yoga entails diving into its complex philosophy and embracing its transforming practice. The idea of yoga encourages us to understand our connectivity and tap into the holy spirit within us.

The practice of yoga gives a vehicle to embody these teachings, creating bodily health, mental clarity, and spiritual progress. As people engage on the journey of philosophy and practice, they expose themselves to the deep and timeless knowledge of yoga, adopting a path of self-realisation and embracing a life of purpose and meaning.

THE EIGHT LIMBS OF YOGA: EMBRACING A HOLISTIC PATH TOWARDS WHOLENESS

Yoga, with its ancient roots and ageless wisdom, provides a complete and holistic approach to living a meaningful and satisfying life. At the centre of this transforming journey lies the Eight Limbs of Yoga, a complex system of ethical and spiritual principles that lead practitioners toward physical well-being, mental clarity, and spiritual revelation.

This holistic approach covers all parts of the human experience, integrating the body, mind, and soul in a beautiful dance toward completeness.
Yamas (Restraints):

The first limb, Yamas, contains a set of ethical rules that regulate our conduct and relationships with the world around us. It contains non-violence (ahimsa), honesty (satya), non-stealing (asteya), moderation (brahmacharya), and non-possessiveness (aparigraha). By embracing these values, we create compassion, honesty, and satisfaction, cultivating harmonious relationships and a feeling of oneness with all living creatures.

Niyamas (Observances): The second limb, Niyamas, focuses on personal observances and self-discipline. It comprises purity (saucha), contentment (santosha), self-discipline (tapas), self-study (svadhyaya), and submission to a higher power (ishvara pranidhana). By exercising Niyamas, we cleanse our inner world, develop gratitude, and improve our awareness of the self, eventually creating a feeling of submission to the greater wisdom that leads us.

Asanas (Postures): The third limb, Asanas, refers to the physical postures done in yoga. While frequently the most obvious component of yoga, Asanas have a deeper purpose beyond physical conditioning. They promote strength, flexibility, and balance in the body, preparing it for the deeper practices of meditation and interior investigation. Asanas also enhance mindfulness and present-moment awareness as we proceed through each position with conscious breath.

Pranayama (Breath Control): The fourth limb, Pranayama, incorporates breathwork methods that harness the life force energy (prana) inside the body. Pranayama techniques soothe the mind, relieve stress, and vitalize the body. By actively managing the breath, practitioners synchronise the body and mind, providing the door for deeper levels of meditation and inner serenity.

Pratyahara (Withdrawal of the Senses): The fifth limb, Pratyahara, is the practice of going within by withdrawing the senses from outward distractions. In a world overwhelmed with sensory inputs, Pratyahara helps us to concentrate our attention on our inner world, quieting the mind and fostering a deep state of introspection.

Dharana (attention): The sixth limb, Dharana, entails establishing steady attention on a single point or object. Through concentrated attention, we teach the mind to stay stable, free from distractions. Dharana prepares the mind for the next level of meditation, enabling us to dig deeper into the depths of awareness.

Dhyana (Meditation): The seventh limb, Dhyana, is the condition of continuous contemplation when the mind is entirely engrossed in the object of meditation. In Dhyana, the practitioner feels a deep sensation of inner serenity, clarity, and heightened self-awareness. This meditative state creates a profound connection with the inner self and universal awareness.

Samadhi (Union):
The eighth and final limb, Samadhi, symbolises the ultimate objective of yoga — a condition of

transcendence and unity with the universal consciousness. In Samadhi, the practitioner has a deep revelation of the interconnection of all things, transcending the limits of the human ego. It is a state of tremendous happiness, insight, and release.

The Eight Limbs of Yoga, considered collectively, create a complete and transforming route towards wholeness, directing practitioners towards physical health, mental clarity, emotional balance, and spiritual enlightenment.

Embracing this holistic approach, we go on a path of self-discovery and self-mastery, integrating the body, mind, and soul in harmony with the universal awareness that flows through all of creation.

THE ROLE OF ASANAS (POSTURES) IN YOGA THERAPY

THE SCIENCE BEHIND YOGA THERAPY

Yoga Therapy, an emerging area within the sphere of healthcare, bridges the gap between ancient yogic knowledge and current scientific understanding.

While the foundations of yoga stretch back thousands of years, modern scientific study has started to expose the practical and evidence-based advantages of yoga on physical, mental, and emotional well-being.

 The synthesis of these traditional traditions with current scientific findings provides the cornerstone of the science underpinning Yoga Therapy.
Neurological Impact:

Modern neuroscience has given insight into the neurological changes that occur in the brain during yoga practice. Studies employing brain imaging methods, such as fMRI and EEG, have demonstrated that yoga and meditation practices activate multiple brain areas important for emotion control, attention, memory, and self-awareness. Regular yoga practice has been related to increased grey matter volume, which is connected with enhanced cognitive abilities and emotional resilience.

Stress Reduction and the Relaxation Response: One of the most well-established advantages of yoga is its ability to lower stress and activate the relaxation response.

Yoga activities, especially breathwork (pranayama) and mindfulness meditation have been demonstrated to reduce cortisol levels, the hormone linked with stress. By engaging the parasympathetic nervous system, yoga generates a state of calm and enhances the body's natural healing capabilities.

Psychoneuroimmunology: The area of psychoneuroimmunology studies the link between the mind, neurological system, and immune system. Research reveals that yoga and meditation activities effectively benefit the immune system by lowering inflammation and boosting immunological function. This link between mind and body shows the promise of yoga therapy in boosting general health and immunological resistance.

Endocrine System Regulation:

The endocrine system, responsible for hormone production and control, is altered by yoga practices. Certain yoga postures and breathwork methods have been demonstrated to alter hormone levels, notably stress-related chemicals like cortisol and adrenaline. This hormonal balance leads to increased emotional well-being and metabolic health.

Pain Management: Yoga therapy has demonstrated potential effects in addressing chronic pain issues. Studies show that regular yoga practice helps decrease pain by raising pain tolerance, lowering pain-related stress, and enhancing overall quality of life. Yoga's emphasis on gentle movements, stretching, and relaxing adds to its success as a non-pharmacological pain treatment method.

Cardiovascular Health: Yoga's influence on cardiovascular health has gained substantial attention. Research suggests that yoga activities, especially asanas, and pranayama, may decrease blood pressure, enhance heart rate variability, and reduce cardiovascular risk factors. These results underscore the possibility of yoga therapy as a supplemental approach to heart health.

Emotional Regulation and Mental Well-being: Yoga therapy has been widely examined for its good impact on mental health. Regular practice has been related to decreased symptoms of anxiety, sadness, and post-traumatic stress disorder (PTSD). Yoga's focus on mindfulness, self-compassion, and emotional control adds to its efficacy as a therapeutic technique for mental well-being.

Enhancing Cognitive Function: Yoga's influence on cognitive function and brain health has been a focus of attention in recent studies. Evidence shows that regular yoga practice may boost cognitive capacities such as attention, memory, and executive function. These results hint at the possibility of yoga therapy as a supplemental method for persons wishing to enhance cognitive function.

In conclusion, the research underpinning yoga therapy reveals the deep and concrete effects of these ancient practices on physical, mental, and emotional well-being. Modern research has uncovered the neurological, physiological, and psychological changes that occur during yoga practice, verifying its therapeutic potential. The blending of ancient yogic knowledge with current scientific understanding has given birth to a comprehensive and evidence-based approach to health and healing, making yoga therapy an increasingly recognized and regarded technique within the field of healthcare.

THE MIND-BODY CONNECTION: HOW YOGA AFFECTS THE BRAIN AND NERVOUS SYSTEM

Yoga Therapy techniques such as magnetic resonance imaging (MRI), have indicated that yoga practitioners demonstrate higher grey matter volume in brain areas related to memory, learning, and emotional control. These changes are especially obvious in regions such as the hippocampus and prefrontal cortex, which play essential roles in cognitive skills and emotional well-being.

Neurotransmitter Regulation:
Yoga techniques, particularly breathwork (pranayama) and meditation alter neurotransmitter activity in the brain. Research reveals that yoga boosts the synthesis of gamma-aminobutyric acid (GABA), a neurotransmitter that promotes relaxation and decreases anxiety. Increased GABA levels contribute to a soothing impact on the neurological system, helping to reduce stress and enhance emotional stability.

Additionally, yoga has been related to the release of endorphins, the brain's natural pain-relieving and mood-enhancing chemicals. These neurochemical changes lead to the emotions of well-being and happiness frequently experienced during and after a yoga session.

Autonomic Nervous System Balance: The autonomic nervous system (ANS) governs involuntary body activities, including heart rate, digestion, and breathing. It consists of two branches: the sympathetic nervous system (SNS), responsible for the "fight or flight" reaction, and the parasympathetic nervous system (PNS), responsible for the "rest and digest" response.

Yoga activities, especially relaxation methods, and breathwork, stimulate the PNS, causing the relaxation response and lowering the activity of the SNS. This change towards parasympathetic dominance promotes a state of tranquillity, decreases stress hormones like cortisol, and boosts the body's capacity to repair and recover.

Mindfulness and Enhanced Brain Function: The practice of mindfulness, a key part of yoga, includes being completely present in the moment without judgement. Mindfulness meditation, commonly included in yoga practices, has been demonstrated to boost brain function and cognitive ability.

Studies employing functional MRI (fMRI) have demonstrated that mindfulness meditation enhances activity in brain areas related to attention, concentration, and cognitive control. Regular practice enhances sustained attention and working memory, making people more competent at handling stress, making choices, and processing information.

Emotion Regulation and Resilience: Yoga's effect on emotional regulation and resilience is strongly connected to its effect on the brain. As yoga increases neuroplasticity and neurotransmitter balance, people may feel enhanced emotional control and higher emotional resilience.

Practitioners generally report decreased sensations of anxiety, despair, and emotional reactivity following continuous yoga practice. The mix of attentive awareness, breathwork, and physical postures cultivates a feeling of emotional balance and helps people to react to life's obstacles with equanimity.

In conclusion, the mind-body link sits at the foundation of yoga's significant influence on the brain and neurological system. Through its effect on neuroplasticity, neurotransmitter activity, and autonomic nervous system balance, yoga develops physical and mental well-being. By adopting mindfulness and boosting brain function, yoga helps people to handle life's difficulties with resilience, clarity, and emotional stability.

As scientific study continues to disclose the nuances of the mind-body link, yoga remains a powerful tool for improving holistic health and embracing the intrinsic capacity for development and change inside each person.

PSYCHONEUROIMMUNOLOGY AND YOGA THERAPY

Psychoneuroimmunology (PNI) is an interdisciplinary subject that examines the delicate link between the mind, the neurological system, and the immune system. This growing field of study has shed light on the tremendous influence of psychological and emotional elements on the immune response and general health. Yoga therapy, with its holistic approach to well-being, connects beautifully with PMI principles, delivering a complementary and evidence-based method to boost the immune system and increase general health.
The Mind-Body Connection in PNI:

PNI acknowledges the interdependence of psychological, neurological, and immunological processes inside the body. Stress, emotions, and mental states may alter the neurological system and hormonal balance, eventually compromising immune function. For example, persistent stress may lead to the production of stress hormones, such as cortisol, which decrease immune function and increase vulnerability to sickness.

Conversely, happy emotional states, relaxation, and mindfulness techniques have been proven to influence the immune response favourably.

When people experience happy emotions and participate in behaviours that promote relaxation, the body creates neuropeptides and neurotransmitters that support immune function and general health.
Yoga Therapy and the Immune System:

Yoga therapy provides a complete approach to promoting well-being by treating physical, mental, and emotional components of health. By adopting yoga practices that promote relaxation, mindfulness, and stress reduction, people may favourably affect their immune systems and nurture optimum health.
Stress Reduction:

One of the primary advantages of yoga therapy is its capacity to alleviate tension and promote relaxation. The practice of yoga, comprising asanas (physical postures), pranayama (breathwork), and meditation, stimulates the parasympathetic nerve system, generating a relaxation response. This, in turn, inhibits the synthesis of stress hormones, such as cortisol, and promotes immunological function.

Mindfulness and immunological Resilience: Mindfulness techniques, a core component of yoga therapy, promote immunological resilience by lowering stress-induced inflammation. Mindfulness meditation and mindful activity foster present-moment awareness, which helps minimise the detrimental effects of stress on the immune system.

Enhanced Emotional Well-being: Yoga therapy encourages emotional well-being by developing self-awareness, self-compassion, and emotional control. By identifying and processing emotions healthily, people may minimise emotional discomfort and boost immunological function.

Movement and Lymphatic Flow: Physical movement in yoga therapy, especially gentle and flowing practices, stimulates lymphatic circulation. The lymphatic system plays a critical role in immunological function by eliminating toxins and waste products from the body. Regular yoga practice helps promote lymphatic flow, therefore aiding the body's immunological response.
Breathwork and immunological Modulation: Pranayama, or breath control techniques, regulate the autonomic nervous system, which, in turn, affects immunological function. Specific pranayama practices, such as alternate nostril breathing, have been demonstrated to modulate immunological responses and balance the body's physiological functions.

Coping with Chronic Illness: For persons suffering from chronic diseases or autoimmune problems, yoga therapy provides a helpful and empowering approach. By treating both the physical and mental components of health, yoga therapy may enhance the overall quality of life and assist the body's natural healing processes.

Psychoneuroimmunology concepts with yoga treatment reveals the great potential of the mind-body link in promoting immune function and general well-being. By mixing stress reduction strategies, mindfulness practices, gentle movement, and breathwork, yoga therapy offers a comprehensive approach to increasing immunological resilience and supporting optimum health. As scientific study continues to examine the fundamental relationships between the mind,
neurological system, and immune system, yoga therapy is a powerful and evidence-based technique for promoting.

YOGA THERAPY FOR PHYSICAL HEALTH

Yoga therapy, a specialist application of yoga concepts and practices, provides a comprehensive approach to enhancing physical health and well-being. By adopting personalised yoga practices and adjustments, people may treat a broad variety of physical issues, facilitate healing, and boost overall physical well-being. From treating chronic pain to developing flexibility and strength, yoga therapy encourages people to take an active part in their health and recovery journey.

Managing Chronic Pain:

Chronic pain disorders, such as lower back pain, arthritis, and fibromyalgia, may greatly influence one's quality of life. Yoga therapy is a gentle and effective method of alleviating chronic pain. Specific yoga postures and motions may help release stress, enhance flexibility, and strengthen muscles to support the afflicted regions.

Breathwork and relaxation practices integrated into yoga therapy sessions help pain reduction by triggering the body's relaxation response and soothing the nervous system. Over time, persistent yoga therapy practice may lead to better pain management and a stronger feeling of control over one's physical well-being.

Enhancing Flexibility and Mobility: Regular yoga practice is well-known for its ability to promote flexibility and joint mobility. Yoga therapy takes this a step further by adapting practices to the individual's particular demands and physical condition.
By carefully and progressively going through modest stretches and motions, people may enhance their joint range of motion and improve overall flexibility. Yoga treatment also targets muscular imbalances, helping to restore balance and function in the body.
Improving Strength and Stability:

Yoga treatment employs different yoga postures and bodyweight exercises to enhance strength and stability. The emphasis on activating core muscles and maintaining good alignment throughout poses helps to strengthen the muscles that support the spine and joints.

For persons healing from accidents or surgery, yoga therapy offers a gentle and safe method to improve strength and regain stability. Props and adaptations are utilised as required to meet individual talents and restrictions. Promoting Balance and Fall Prevention:
Balance difficulties and the fear of falling are typical concerns, particularly among older persons. Yoga

treatment incorporates balance-enhancing techniques that increase proprioception (awareness of body position in space) and stability.

Standing postures and particular balancing exercises assist people build more stability and confidence in their actions. This may be especially advantageous for elderly persons or those with neurological problems that impact balance.

Supporting Cardiovascular Health: Certain kinds of yoga therapy, such as mild flow sequences and heart-opening poses, may promote cardiovascular health. These routines promote circulation, boost heart rate variability, and contribute to overall cardiovascular fitness.

Yoga treatment also focuses on breathwork, which has a direct influence on the cardiovascular system by inducing relaxation, decreasing blood pressure, and improving oxygenation.

Enhancing Posture and Body Awareness: Modern lives can lead to poor posture and muscle imbalances, which may contribute to pain and discomfort. Yoga treatment promotes body awareness and good alignment in daily motions.

By promoting awareness of posture and alignment, people become more cognizant of how they hold their bodies and move throughout the day. This heightened awareness may lead to better posture and less strain on the musculoskeletal system.

In conclusion, yoga therapy provides a customised and comprehensive approach to increasing physical health and well-being. Through a mix of particular yoga postures, breathwork, relaxation methods, and mindfulness practices, people may manage chronic pain, increase flexibility, strength, and balance, and enhance overall physical well-being. Whether treating particular physical ailments or looking to promote general vitality, yoga therapy encourages people to take ownership of their health and create a deeper connection with their bodies.

YOGA THERAPY FOR MUSCULOSKELETAL HEALTH

Yoga therapy provides a specific and successful method for resolving musculoskeletal disorders and improving the optimum health of the muscles, bones, and joints. By integrating the ancient wisdom of yoga with the current understanding of anatomy and biomechanics, yoga therapy tackles particular musculoskeletal disorders, develops flexibility, and improves general musculoskeletal function. Whether suffering from chronic pain, injury rehabilitation, or just looking to maintain a healthy musculoskeletal system, yoga therapy offers a thorough and holistic approach.

Managing Chronic Pain: Chronic musculoskeletal pain, such as back pain, neck pain, and joint pain, may profoundly impair everyday living. Yoga treatment focuses on gentle and precise movements to reduce pain and discomfort. Specific yoga poses, such as moderate stretches, twists, and backbends, help relieve tension, enhance flexibility, and strengthen the supporting muscles surrounding the problematic regions.

Breathwork and relaxation practices integrated into yoga therapy sessions assist alleviate pain by increasing calm and lowering tension, which frequently exacerbates musculoskeletal pain.

Improving Posture and Alignment: Poor posture and misalignments may contribute to musculoskeletal imbalances and discomfort. Yoga treatment promotes body awareness and good alignment in daily motions.
Through individualised yoga sequences and alignment cues, people become more cognizant of their posture and body mechanics. This heightened awareness helps rectify imbalances and aids the body in maintaining good alignment.

Enhancing Flexibility and Joint Health: Regular yoga practice is famous for its ability to promote flexibility and joint mobility. Yoga therapy goes this further by adapting practices to individual requirements and limitations.

Gentle stretches and joint-specific exercises in yoga therapy increase the joint range of motion and decrease stiffness. This may be especially useful for persons with diseases like arthritis or those recuperating from trauma.
Strengthening Muscles and Stability: Yoga treatment involves a range of yoga postures and bodyweight exercises to strengthen the muscles that support the musculoskeletal system. Emphasis is centred on

activating core muscles and engaging stabilising muscles to develop strength and stability.

Individualised yoga therapy sessions take into consideration individual talents and limits, guaranteeing safe and effective strengthening techniques.
Injury Healing and Rehabilitation: Yoga therapy offers a gentle and supportive approach to injury healing and rehabilitation. Individuals recuperating from musculoskeletal ailments might benefit from specialised yoga sequences that help in healing, restore mobility, and minimise additional tension on the damaged regions.

Yoga treatment also increases mindfulness and body awareness, enabling patients to tune into their body's signals and prevent overexertion throughout the rehabilitation process.

Enhancing Overall Musculoskeletal Function: Beyond treating particular disorders, yoga therapy attempts to promote overall musculoskeletal function. By using a well-rounded blend of yoga postures, breathwork, and relaxation methods, yoga therapy enhances the entire health and vitality of the musculoskeletal system.
This complete strategy helps people maintain joint health, minimise the likelihood of accidents, and enhance overall physical performance.

In conclusion, yoga therapy provides a tailored and integrated approach to musculoskeletal health, treating individual difficulties and boosting general well-being. By integrating the wisdom of yoga with current knowledge of anatomy and biomechanics, yoga therapy tackles chronic pain, improves flexibility, alignment, and stability, and promotes injury healing and rehabilitation. Whether struggling with musculoskeletal issues or just trying to increase general physical health, yoga therapy encourages people to move consciously, heal, and strengthen their bodies, supporting optimum musculoskeletal function and overall vitality.

ADDRESSING CHRONIC PAIN AND INJURIES THROUGH YOGA

Chronic pain and injuries may be devastating, hurting one's quality of life and general well-being. Yoga, with its gentle but powerful approach, provides an effective and comprehensive technique to relieve chronic pain and promote the healing process for injuries. By combining certain yoga practices, people may find relief, enhance mobility, and create a deeper feeling of body awareness and self-empowerment.

Gentle Movement and Pain Relief: Yoga treatment for chronic pain and injuries frequently starts with gentle movements and postures adapted to the individual's condition. Gentle stretching and range-of-motion exercises can release muscular tension, decrease stiffness, and alleviate discomfort.

Yoga's concentration on breath awareness also plays a key impact in pain reduction. By employing breathwork (pranayama) and mindful breathing practices, people may relax the body and soothe the neurological system, lowering the severity of pain feelings.

Targeted Strengthening: Yoga treatment combines targeted strengthening exercises to assist damaged regions and enhance overall musculoskeletal function. These workouts are customised to meet the individual's demands and restrictions.

The activation of core muscles and stabilising muscles helps distribute the weight more evenly throughout the body, decreasing tension in affected regions. Strengthening the surrounding muscles also assists in avoiding future injuries and offers stronger support throughout the healing process.

Mindfulness and Pain Management: Central to yoga therapy is the practice of mindfulness, which helps people to be completely present and sensitive to their bodies. This heightened awareness helps people to detect pain triggers, pinpoint regions of tension, and make modifications to decrease suffering.

Mindfulness activities, including meditation and body scanning, may help patients build a new connection with pain, lessening the emotional anguish commonly linked with chronic pain and injury.

Flexibility and Range of Motion: Yoga postures and motions increase flexibility and better range of motion, which may be particularly useful for persons coping with stiffness and limited mobility due to injuries.

By progressively going through moderate stretches and joint-specific exercises, people may improve joint mobility and enhance flexibility, assisting in the healing process and lowering the chance of additional injuries.

Tension Reduction and Relaxation: Chronic pain and injuries may frequently lead to heightened tension and anxiety. Yoga therapy's focus on relaxation methods and stress reduction may considerably aid persons suffering from pain.
Relaxation therapies, such as guided imagery and progressive muscle relaxation, produce a relaxation response, soothing the body and mind, and helping to manage pain more effectively.

Building Self-Empowerment: Yoga therapy creates a feeling of self-empowerment by encouraging people to take an active part in their recovery path. Through individualised practices, people get a better awareness of their bodies and become more attentive to their specific needs and talents.

The feeling of control and agency established by yoga therapy may enhance confidence and give a positive attitude throughout the healing process.

In conclusion, yoga offers a diverse and compassionate approach to healing chronic pain and injury. By combining gentle movements, focused strengthening, mindfulness, and stress reduction methods, yoga therapy helps the body's natural healing processes and increases general well-being. Whether seeking relief from chronic pain or recuperating from an accident, yoga therapy allows patients to embrace their healing path, establish balance, and rediscover a feeling of completeness and self-empowerment.

ENHANCING FLEXIBILITY, BALANCE, AND POSTURE THROUGH YOGA

Yoga, with its centuries-old heritage of fostering physical and mental well-being, provides a holistic approach to strengthening flexibility, balance, and posture. By integrating dynamic asanas (postures), breathwork, and mindfulness techniques, people may begin on a transformational path toward physical mastery and conscious alignment.

Flexibility: Yoga is recognized for its ability to promote flexibility and joint mobility. Through a systematic and gentle approach, yoga poses and stretches progressively enhance flexibility in muscles and connective tissues.

Dynamic and static stretching methods in yoga serve to lengthen and release tight muscles, minimising the risk of injury and boosting general flexibility. Consistent yoga practice creates an expanded range of motion, enabling people to move with more ease and fluidity.

Balance: Yoga includes balance-enhancing activities to build stability and proprioception (awareness of body position in space). Standing postures test balance and build strength in stabilising muscles.

Balancing poses like Tree Pose (Vrksasana) and Warrior III (Virabhadrasana III) demand attention and concentration, helping people to discover equilibrium both on and off the mat. Enhanced balance enhances coordination and stability, minimising the chance of falls and accidents.

Posture: Yoga lays tremendous emphasis on mindful alignment and body awareness, which directly affects posture. By practising yoga poses with optimal alignment, people build improved postural habits in everyday life.

Yoga therapy sessions frequently incorporate alignment instructions to assist clients maintain a neutral spine and activate core muscles. Consistent practice strengthens these good postural habits, minimising pressure on the spine and improving general musculoskeletal health.
Core Strength: The core muscles play a critical role in strengthening flexibility, balance, and posture. Yoga contains several postures that activate and develop the core, such as Plank Pose (Phalakasana) and Boat Pose (Navasana).

A strong core stabilises the spine and pelvis, providing a sturdy basis for the body's motions. It also helps good alignment and posture, leading to a healthier and more robust musculoskeletal system.

Mindfulness and Body Awareness:
The mind-body link in yoga creates heightened bodily awareness and mindfulness. By concentrating on the breath and feelings during yoga practice, people become more sensitive to their bodies' demands and limits.
Mindful movement promotes people to move with purpose and presence, lowering the danger of overextending or straining during yoga poses. This heightened awareness spills over into everyday life, fostering attentive movement and healthier postural habits.

Breathwork for Relaxation: Yoga utilises breathwork (pranayama) to promote relaxation and relieve tension. Deep and regulated breathing relaxes the nervous system, helping people to achieve peace and relaxation in hard positions.

Relaxed breathing during yoga practice stimulates muscular relaxation and enables the body to open up to better flexibility and balance. Moreover, breath awareness throughout the day helps manage stress and promotes improved posture and body alignment.

In conclusion, yoga provides a transforming route to developing flexibility, balance, and posture. Through conscious alignment, strengthening core muscles, and fostering body awareness, people may experience enhanced flexibility, stability, and total physical mastery.

Yoga's comprehensive approach to well-being goes beyond the mat, encouraging people to incorporate mindfulness and body consciousness into their everyday lives. With persistent practice and devotion, yoga becomes a powerful instrument for embracing physical and mental harmony, fostering a lifetime journey towards improved flexibility, balance, and conscious alignment.

YOGA FOR CARDIOVASCULAR AND RESPIRATORY HEALTH

YOGA THERAPY FOR MENTAL HEALTH

Yoga therapy provides a deep and comprehensive approach to boosting mental health and emotional well-being. By blending yoga practices with concepts of psychology and mindfulness, yoga therapy tackles a broad variety of mental health disorders, from stress and anxiety to depression and trauma. Through breathwork, mindful movement, and meditation, people may grow self-awareness, emotional regulation, and resilience, helping them to discover balance and healing in their mental and emotional domains.

Stress Reduction and Anxiety Management: Yoga therapy's focus on breathwork (pranayama) and relaxation methods aids stress reduction and anxiety management. By stimulating the body's relaxation response, yoga therapy helps soothe the nervous system, lowering stress chemicals like cortisol and generating a feeling of serenity and tranquillity.

Mindful movement in yoga therapy helps patients shift their attention from worried thoughts to the present moment, relieving anxiety and building a stronger feeling of control over their emotional states.

Emotional Regulation: Yoga therapy allows people to examine their emotions in a safe and non-judgmental atmosphere. Through mindfulness activities, people may acquire better emotional awareness and learn to manage their experiences with compassion and understanding.

Practices such as yoga nidra (a guided meditation for deep relaxation) and loving-kindness meditation encourage self-compassion and empathy, helping people create stronger connections with themselves and others.

Depression Management: Yoga therapy may be a beneficial technique in controlling depression by addressing both the physical and emotional elements of the disorder. Gentle and restorative yoga poses help ease physical stress and exhaustion typically linked with sadness.

Breath-centred activities in yoga therapy boost mood and energy levels by enhancing oxygenation and fostering a feeling of vigour. Furthermore, yoga's mind-body connection develops a feeling of empowerment and optimism, crucial for people coping with depression.

Trauma recovery: For persons struggling with trauma, yoga therapy provides a gentle and supportive approach to recovery. Yoga routines are tailored to provide safety and prevent evoking unpleasant memories.

Yoga therapy offers a place for people to reconnect with their bodies and process their experiences carefully. Mindful movement and breathwork help the release of accumulated stress, supporting healing on a somatic level.

Mindfulness for Mental Clarity: Mindfulness techniques are a cornerstone of yoga therapy, fostering mental clarity and presence. By training the mind to concentrate on the present moment without judgement, people may lessen ruminative thinking and break free from cycles of negative ideas.

Mindfulness meditation and body scanning activities help anchor the mind in the here and now, generating a feeling of tranquillity and mental clarity.

Self-Reflection and Personal Growth: Yoga therapy emphasises self-reflection and introspection. Journaling and guided self-inquiry activities help people investigate their ideas, emotions, and actions, offering insights into patterns and opportunities for personal improvement.

Yoga therapy sessions may become a place for self-discovery, helping people to expand their awareness of themselves and encourage good changes in their life.

In conclusion, yoga therapy acts as an effective and caring technique for promoting mental health and emotional well-being. By combining breathwork, mindful movement, and meditation, people may build emotional control, decrease stress and anxiety, and find healing from trauma and despair. Yoga therapy helps people to embrace the mind-body connection, building self-awareness, resilience, and a greater feeling of self-compassion. As a supplementary approach to mental health treatment, yoga therapy offers the potential to induce remarkable shifts, assisting people on their path toward emotional balance and general well-being.

YOGA'S IMPACT ON MENTAL WELL-BEING

Yoga, with its ancient roots and deep knowledge, delivers a transforming influence on mental well-being. Through a comprehensive approach that incorporates physical postures, breathwork, meditation, and mindfulness practices, yoga improves emotional balance, decreases stress, and nourishes a deeper feeling of inner calm.

Whether coping with regular stress or managing mental health concerns, yoga offers a strong tool for increasing mental well-being and building a harmonious mind-body connection.

Stress Reduction and Relaxation: One of the most well-known advantages of yoga is its ability to relieve stress and promote relaxation. Yoga activities, such as deep breathing exercises (pranayama) and restorative postures, stimulate the body's relaxation response, relaxing the nervous system and lowering stress chemicals like cortisol.

Regular practice of yoga assists people to build better coping skills for dealing with stress, allowing them to handle life's problems with more equanimity.

Emotional control: Yoga improves emotional control by teaching people to notice and accept their feelings without judgement. Through mindfulness activities, people may grow better emotional awareness and create healthier ways of reacting to their experiences.
The practice of mindfulness meditation helps people to view thoughts and feelings as fleeting occurrences, lowering reactivity and boosting emotional resilience.

Anxiety and Depression Management: Studies have indicated that yoga may be effective in treating anxiety and depression. Yoga's mind-body approach tackles both the physical and emotional elements of these illnesses.

Yoga poses and movement reduce physical stress and stimulate the flow of good energy, leading to an improved mood. The concentration on breath awareness and meditation calms the mind and lowers ruminating, frequent anxiety, and depression.

Increased Self-awareness: Yoga improves self-awareness by encouraging people to listen to their bodies and thoughts. By practising mindful movement and reflection, people obtain deeper insights into their thoughts, habits, and routines.

Increased self-awareness helps people to make mindful decisions and create a better feeling of self-compassion and acceptance.

Enhanced Cognitive Function: Yoga's influence on mental well-being extends to cognitive function. Mindfulness techniques, such as focused attention during yoga postures and meditation, boost cognitive capacities, including attention, memory, and executive function.

Regular yoga practice has been connected with enhanced cognitive function and increased brain connection, leading to mental clarity and cognitive resilience.

Cultivation of Inner calm: At its foundation, yoga attempts to create inner calm and satisfaction. By connecting with the present moment and adopting the practice of non-attachment, people may feel a sense of calm that transcends external circumstances.

Yoga philosophy includes notions like Ahimsa (non-violence) and Santosha (contentment), which urges people to discover peace within themselves and in their interactions with others.

In conclusion, yoga's influence on mental well-being is extensive and diverse. By managing stress, increasing emotional control, and building self-awareness and inner serenity, yoga acts as a great tool for boosting mental well-being and strengthening the mind-body connection.

The transforming power of yoga rests in its potential to enable people to take responsibility for their mental health and embrace a path of balance, resilience, and inner peace. Whether as a supplemental approach to mental health treatment or as a practice for general well-being, yoga provides a path toward increased mental clarity, emotional stability, and a more deep connection to oneself and the world around us.

MANAGING STRESS AND ANXIETY WITH YOGA TECHNIQUES

Stress and anxiety are widespread issues in contemporary life, impacting mental and physical well-being. Yoga, with its comprehensive approach to health, gives helpful techniques to reduce stress and anxiety. By combining certain yoga methods, people may find relief, develop peace, and build resilience in the face of life's pressures. The following yoga poses are especially effective for reducing stress and anxiety:
Deep Breathing (Pranayama):

Pranayama, or breath control methods, provide the core of stress and anxiety treatment in yoga. Deep breathing stimulates the parasympathetic nerve system, prompting the body's relaxation response and lowering the "fight or flight" stress reaction.

One powerful pranayama method is the 4-7-8 breath: Inhale for a count of 4, hold the breath for a count of 7, and exhale for a count of 8. Practising this method multiple times a day will help relax the mind and lessen worry.

Mindful Movement (Asanas): Yoga postures (asanas) are recognized for their ability to alleviate physical tension and induce relaxation. Gentle, flowing movements assist to release built-up tension in the body and relax the mind.

Practising grounding poses, such as Child's Pose (Balasana) and Legs-Up-the-Wall (Viparita Karani), may be especially relaxing during times of stress and worry.

Yoga Nidra (Yogic Sleep): Yoga Nidra is a guided meditation practice that generates a state of profound relaxation, akin to the moments shortly before falling asleep. This technique helps decrease stress and anxiety by soothing the nervous system and releasing tension.

During Yoga Nidra, participants are taken through a methodical process of body awareness, breathwork, and imagery, promoting deep relaxation and regeneration.

Mindfulness Meditation: Mindfulness meditation includes concentrating attention on the present moment without judgement. By noticing thoughts and feelings as they emerge, people acquire a non-reactive and accepting approach toward stress and worry.

Consistent mindfulness meditation practice helps generate space from worrying thoughts and promotes a stronger feeling of inner serenity.

Progressive Muscle Calm: Progressive Muscle Relaxation (PMR) is a method that includes tensing and then releasing various muscle groups to produce physical and mental calm. PMR helps people notice and release body tension, a frequent indicator of stress and anxiety.

By systematically relaxing muscle regions, PMR may bring about a deep sensation of relaxation and alleviation from stress-induced physical tension.

Cultivating Gratitude and Self-Compassion: Yoga teaches the practice of gratitude and self-compassion as a technique to alleviate stress and anxiety. Gratitude activities, such as maintaining a gratitude diary, shift emphasis from what is missing to what is there and cultivating a good mindset.

Self-compassion techniques entail treating oneself with care and empathy, particularly during stressful circumstances. This builds resilience and a feeling of inner support.

In conclusion, yoga provides some helpful strategies to manage stress and anxiety, increasing mental and emotional well-being. By integrating deep breathing, mindful movement, guided relaxation, meditation, and developing appreciation and self-compassion, people may construct a toolbox of practices to handle stress with more ease. Regular yoga practice not only helps handle current pressures but also improves resilience, helping people to tackle life's obstacles with enhanced peace, balance, and self-awareness.

YOGA FOR DEPRESSION AND MOOD DISORDERS

Depression and mood disorders may significantly damage one's emotional well-being, making it tough to find respite and maintain inner balance. Yoga, with its mind-body approach, provides a complementary and powerful technique to help persons struggling with these illnesses. By integrating breathwork, yoga postures, meditation, and self-compassion practices, yoga may play a crucial role in reducing depression symptoms, encouraging emotional healing, and restoring a feeling of inner peace.

Mindful Movement and Mood Elevation: Yoga's mindful movement helps boost mood by stimulating the production of endorphins, the body's natural mood enhancers. Flowing sequences and dynamic postures ignite the body's energy, reducing feelings of lethargy and exhaustion typically linked with sadness.
The concentration on breath synchronisation while exercise cultivates a feeling of presence, anchoring persons in the here and now, minimising rumination and negative thinking patterns.

Breath-Centred Practices for Emotional Control: Breath-centred practices, such as pranayama, provide a strong tool for emotional control. Specific breathing practices, such as the Three-Part Breath (Dirga Pranayama) or Alternate Nostril Breathing (Nadi Shodhana), relax the nervous system and assist in the control of anxiety and depression symptoms.

Conscious and deep breathing stimulates the parasympathetic nervous system, encouraging relaxation and lowering the body's stress reaction.

Yoga Nidra for profound Relaxation: Yoga Nidra, also known as Yogic Sleep, is a guided meditation practice that generates a state of profound relaxation. By methodically relaxing the body and mind, Yoga Nidra helps people relieve emotional stress and discover inner serenity.

Regular practice of Yoga Nidra may assist improve sleep quality, which is typically interrupted in mood disorders, and promote general emotional well-being.

Loving-Kindness Meditation: Loving-Kindness Meditation (Metta Meditation) teaches compassion and self-acceptance. By aiming loving and compassionate intentions towards oneself and others, people establish a more positive and caring connection with themselves.

Depression typically entails emotions of self-criticism and worthlessness.

Loving-Kindness Meditation helps offset these negative self-perceptions, encouraging self-compassion and emotional healing.

Mindfulness Meditation for Resilience:
Mindfulness meditation cultivates the capacity to examine thoughts and emotions with non-judgmental awareness. By establishing space between the person and their ideas, mindfulness promotes resilience and lowers sensitivity to depressed triggers.
Mindfulness techniques allow people to accept their emotions without resistance, developing a healthy way to cope with emotional issues.

Community and Connection: Yoga courses and group sessions create a feeling of community and connection, which may be very useful for persons with depression. Engaging in yoga with others develops a sense of connection and decreases feelings of loneliness.
The support of like-minded persons in a secure and loving setting may inspire optimism and help the healing process.

In conclusion, yoga provides a caring and comprehensive approach to managing depression and mood disorders. By blending mindful movement, breath-centred practices, meditation, and self-compassion strategies, yoga helps people to cultivate emotional healing and restore inner balance.

Regular yoga practice may serve as a complementary tool alongside professional mental health treatment, assisting people in their quest to discover relief from depression symptoms and create a deeper feeling of well-being. Yoga's transforming impact resides in its capacity to promote self-awareness, resilience, and a better connection to oneself and others, fostering emotional healing and enduring good change.

YOGA THERAPY FOR TRAUMA AND POST-TRAUMATIC STRESS

YOGA THERAPY FOR SPECIFIC HEALTH CONDITIONS

Yoga therapy is a diverse and adaptive strategy that may be adjusted to meet various health concerns. It complements traditional medical therapies and promotes overall well-being. Here are some instances of how yoga therapy may be useful for different health conditions:

Back Pain & Spinal Issues: Yoga therapy may help ease back pain and improve spinal health by using moderate stretches and strengthening movements. Postures like Cat-Cow (Marjaryasana-Bitilasana) and Child's Pose (Balasana) may bring relaxation and alleviate tension in the back muscles.

Arthritis: Yoga treatment includes moderate movements and modified postures that enhance joint flexibility and decrease inflammation. Controlled breathwork and meditation may also improve pain management and promote general well-being.

Cardiovascular Conditions: Certain yoga practices, such as mild flow sequences and relaxation methods, may enhance cardiovascular health by decreasing blood pressure and boosting heart rate variability.

Respiratory Disorders: Yoga therapy includes particular breathing techniques like Diaphragmatic Breathing (also known as Belly Breathing) and alternate nostril breathing (Nadi Shodhana) that help enhance lung function and maintain respiratory health.

Digestive illnesses: Yoga treatment combines twisting postures and abdominal compressions that might assist digestion and ease symptoms of digestive illnesses such as irritable bowel syndrome (IBS).

Insomnia and Sleep Disorders: Yoga Nidra and relaxation practices induce deep relaxation, allowing patients with insomnia or sleep disorders to have more comfortable sleep.

Women's Health Issues: Yoga therapy helps treat menstruation irregularities, menopausal symptoms, and reproductive health issues in women. Specific postures and relaxation activities may help ease pain and regulate hormone levels.

Mental Health Conditions: As previously indicated, yoga therapy may be useful in controlling stress, anxiety, depression, and other mood disorders by integrating mindful movement, breathwork, and meditation.

Neurological illnesses: Yoga therapy may benefit persons with neurological illnesses such as multiple sclerosis (MS) or Parkinson's disease by concentrating on increasing balance, coordination, and muscular strength.
Post-Traumatic Stress Disorder (PTSD): Yoga therapy includes trauma-sensitive practices that assist persons with PTSD release stored tension in the body and promote emotional resilience via meditation and grounding methods.

Cancer Recovery: Yoga therapy may complement cancer treatment by offering moderate exercise and relaxation activities that enhance physical and mental well-being. It may help lessen medication adverse effects and enhance the quality of life.

It is necessary to work with a qualified yoga therapist or an experienced yoga teacher when employing yoga therapy for certain health concerns. They may customise practices to individual requirements, give necessary changes, and guarantee a safe and supportive atmosphere for healing and well-being.

Additionally, yoga therapy should be implemented as a supplementary strategy with regular medical treatment, engaging with healthcare specialists as appropriate.

YOGA FOR BACK PAIN AND SPINAL HEALTH

Back discomfort and spinal difficulties are typical concerns that may greatly influence everyday living and well-being. Yoga is an effective and comprehensive technique to relieve back pain and enhance spinal health. By adopting certain yoga postures, stretches, and mindful movements, people may strengthen the core, develop flexibility, and find relief from back stiffness. Gentle Stretches for Flexibility: Yoga involves several gentle stretches that enhance flexibility in the back and surrounding muscles. Cat-Cow.

(Marjaryasana-Bitilasana) is a wonderful beginning pose to warm up the spine and enhance its range of motion. Child's Pose (Balasana) is another mild stretch that lengthens the spine and reduces tension in the lower back. Downward Dog (Adho Mukha Svanasana) elongates the whole spine and extends the hamstrings and calves, aiding back pain treatment.

Strengthening the Core and Back Muscles: A strong core and back muscles are necessary for supporting the spine and maintaining good posture. Yoga poses like Boat Pose (Navasana) and Bridge Pose (Setu Bandhasana) activate and develop the core, helping to stabilise the back and relieve pressure on the spine.

Cobra Pose (Bhujangasana) and Locust Pose (Salabhasana) address the muscles of the back, creating strength and flexibility in the whole spinal column.

Spinal Twists for Mobility: Spinal twists are good for preserving spinal mobility and reducing tension in the back. Seated and supine twists, such as Half Lord of the Fishes Pose (Ardha Matsyendrasana) and Supine Spinal Twist (Supta Matsyendrasana), gently rotate the spine, encouraging flexibility and enhancing spinal health.

Supported Inversions for Decompression: Inversions, when the hips are lifted above the heart, may assist decompress the spine and offer relief from back discomfort. Supported versions, such as Legs-Up-the-Wall (Viparita Karani) or Shoulder Stand (Sarvangasana) using supports, are safe possibilities to try with instruction.

Breathwork for Relaxation: Yoga involves breathwork (pranayama) to promote relaxation and decrease stress, which may contribute to back discomfort. Deep breathing methods, like Diaphragmatic Breathing, assist soothe the nervous system and relieve tension in the muscles.

Mindful Movement and Alignment: Mindful movement is a basic part of yoga, encouraging people to move with mindfulness and attention to good alignment. Practising yoga mindfully may help people avoid hurting their backs and establish a healthy connection with movement.

It is vital to approach yoga for back pain with awareness and sensitivity to individual requirements and limits. Consulting with a trained yoga teacher or yoga therapist helps ensure that the practices are adapted to the individual ailment and give necessary adjustments.

Incorporating yoga for back pain as part of a daily self-care regimen may lead to better spine health, enhanced flexibility, and decreased discomfort, boosting overall well-being and increasing the quality of life.

YOGA THERAPY FOR DIGESTIVE DISORDERS

Digestive diseases may cause pain and interrupt normal living. Yoga therapy provides a moderate and comprehensive approach to assist digestive health by using particular yoga techniques that promote relaxation, enhance circulation, and ease digestion. By treating stress, and tension, and establishing attentive eating habits, yoga therapy may be effective for persons living with digestive difficulties. Here are some ways yoga therapy might help:

Breath-Centred Practices:

Breathwork (pranayama) plays a significant part in yoga treatment for digestive issues. Deep abdominal breathing, also known as Diaphragmatic Breathing, engages the parasympathetic nervous system, aiding relaxation and lowering tension. This level of calm facilitates optimum digestion and absorption of nutrients. Gentle Twisting Poses: Yoga treatment involves gentle twisting postures that massage and stimulate the digestive systems. Twists like Seated Spinal Twist (Ardha Matsyendrasana) and Revolved Triangle Pose (Parivrtta Trikonasana) aid to decrease bloating, promote digestion, and relieve pain.

Forward Bends: Forward bending postures, such as Standing Forward Bend (Uttanasana) and Seated Forward Bend (Paschimottanasana), may assist calm the abdomen region and offer a gentle massage to the digestive organs, facilitating improved digestion and excretion.

Relaxation methods: Yoga therapy uses relaxation methods, such as Yoga Nidra and guided meditation, to relieve tension and foster a sense of inner serenity. By controlling stress, people may limit the effect of stress-related digestive disorders, such as irritable bowel syndrome (IBS).

Mindful Eating Activities: Yoga therapy encourages mindful eating activities to aid digestion. Mindful eating entails paying attention to the taste, texture, and scent of food while being present throughout meals. This method promotes digestion by enabling improved chewing and absorption of nutrients.

Abdominal Breathing Exercises: Specific abdominal breathing exercises, including Kapalabhati (Skull Shining Breath), may stimulate the digestive organs and promote peristalsis, the wave-like action that transports food through the digestive system.

Stress Reduction: Chronic stress may aggravate digestive difficulties. Yoga treatment targets stress via relaxation methods, meditation, and gentle movements, promoting overall digestive health.

It is vital to work with a qualified yoga therapist or an experienced yoga teacher when employing yoga therapy for digestive issues. They may customise practices to individual requirements, give necessary changes, and guarantee a safe and supportive atmosphere for healing and well-being.
Yoga therapy provides a comprehensive and compassionate way to cultivate intestinal health. By adding breath-centred practices, mild twisting postures, relaxation methods, and mindful eating habits, people may find relief from digestive pain and create a healthy connection with their digestive system. Consistent yoga treatment may stimulate digestion, reduce symptoms, and boost general well-being.

As with any supplementary approach to health, consumers should check with their healthcare professionals to verify that yoga therapy supports their present medical treatments.

MANAGING DIABETES THROUGH YOGA

Diabetes is a chronic disorder that affects millions of individuals globally. While medical therapy is necessary for controlling diabetes, supplementary techniques like yoga may play a key role in improving blood sugar management, enhancing general well-being, and lowering the risk of complications. Yoga provides a comprehensive approach that includes physical movement, breathwork, stress reduction, and mindful living, encouraging those with diabetes to take an active part in their self-care journey. Here are ways yoga might be good for treating diabetes:

Physical Activity and Insulin Sensitivity:
Regular physical exercise is vital for those with diabetes since it increases insulin sensitivity and helps maintain blood sugar levels. Yoga asanas (postures) provide a mild but effective approach to participate in physical exercise. Practices like Sun Salutations (Surya Namaskar) and Standing Poses (Warrior Pose, Triangle Pose) enhance muscular strength and flexibility, significantly affecting blood glucose levels.

Breathwork (Pranayama) for Stress Management: Stress and high cortisol levels may alter blood sugar levels in patients with diabetes. Pranayama, or breathwork, is a fundamental aspect of yoga that promotes relaxation and decreases tension. Techniques like Diaphragmatic Breathing and Alternate Nostril Breathing assist soothe the nervous system, resulting in improved glycemic control.

Mindful Eating Habits: Yoga emphasises mindful eating habits, which may be particularly useful for those with diabetes. Mindful eating means being completely present throughout meals, paying attention to hunger signals, and relishing each mouthful. This strategy develops a healthy connection with food, helps control portion sizes, and supports improved blood sugar regulation.

Improved Circulation and Nerve Health:
Certain yoga poses, such as Legs-Up-the-Wall (Viparita Karani) and Reclining Bound Angle Pose (Supta Baddha Konasana), promote enhanced blood circulation and neurological health. Better circulation improves the transport of nutrients and oxygen to the body's tissues, while nerve health helps lower the incidence of diabetic neuropathy.

Relaxation methods for Better Sleep: Yoga includes relaxation methods like Yoga Nidra and guided meditation that assist patients with diabetes manage stress and enhance sleep quality. Sufficient restorative sleep is necessary for keeping blood sugar levels within a safe range.

Environment Support and Accountability: Participating in yoga classes or group sessions may create a supportive environment where persons with diabetes can share experiences and learn from one another. This feeling of connection might give incentive and responsibility in controlling the disease.

Persons with diabetes must engage with a trained yoga teacher or yoga therapist who knows the unique demands and limits associated with the illness. They may adjust yoga practices to individual capacities and facilitate the incorporation of yoga into the diabetes care strategy.

Yoga is a wonderful tool for those with diabetes to create more self-awareness, improve blood sugar management, and promote general well-being. By mixing physical movement, breathwork, stress reduction methods, and mindful eating practices, yoga encourages people to take ownership of their health and live with more balance and energy. As with any supplementary approach to health, patients should speak with their healthcare professionals to verify that yoga matches their current diabetes treatment regimen.

CONCLUSION

In the quest of studying the vast domain of yoga therapy, we have embarked on a transforming tour that integrates ancient wisdom with modern science, nourishing the mind, body, and soul. Throughout these pages, we've looked into the delicate interplay between yoga and holistic well-being, uncovering the tremendous potential for healing, development, and self-discovery that this ancient practice possesses.

From the roots of yoga theory to the practical applications of yoga therapy, we've experienced the harmony between breath and movement, the power of mindfulness, and the tenacity of the human spirit. We've investigated the complicated network between the physical body and the mind, discovering how they combine to determine our experiences and impact our health.

Yoga therapy is a testimony to the interconnectedness of mind and body, giving a caring way to resolving a range of health concerns - from physical diseases to emotional difficulties. Through the gentle guidance of yoga's principles, we've unearthed a road towards self-empowerment, acceptance, and a greater awareness of our inner landscapes.

As we complete our trip, let us remember that yoga therapy is not only a collection of methods; it is an invitation to create a healthy connection with ourselves and the world around us. It's a chance to listen to our body, recognize our feelings, and handle life's problems with grace and perseverance.

May this book serve as a source of inspiration, bringing you towards a more meaningful connection with yourself. Whether you're a yoga practitioner, a healthcare professional, or just a seeker of well-being, may the knowledge offered within these pages enable you to begin on a path of healing, self-discovery, and change.

As you continue on your particular road, remember that the adventure of yoga therapy is a lifetime one, full of discoveries and insights. With an open heart and a determined spirit, may you continue to explore the wide geography of your potential, uncovering the riches of well-being, harmony, and inner serenity.